Heat Stroke Management

How to Manage and Prevent Heat Stroke the Right Way

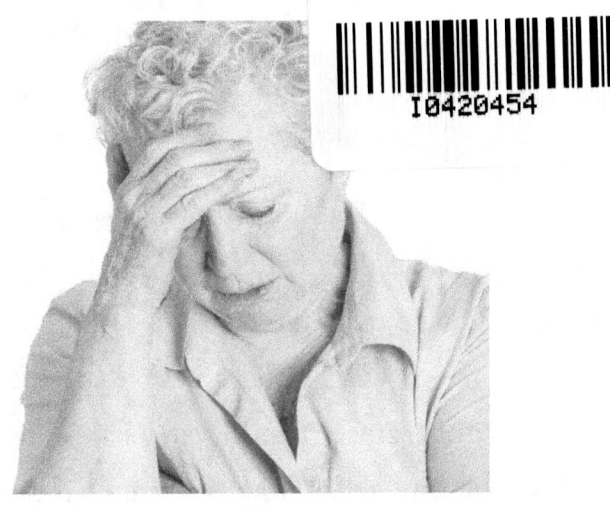

I0420454

By

Paolo Jose de Luna

Paolo Jose De Luna

Paolo Jose De Luna

Paolo Jose De Luna

Table of Contents

INTRODUCTION

Heat is one of the most imposing forces of nature. It's always present, consistently providing us with warmth and comfort, giving us an endearing shelter especially during the colder months. However, heat can become an issue when it is too much.

Water is one of the most basic ways on how to combat heat. With water, the body is cooled down and heat is mitigated to an accepted temperature. The human body is composed of about 70% of water which makes up most of our body. That's the reason why water is essential for our daily needs and it proves to be essential to our survival. This also explains as to why the human body or any living thing for that matter, can't survive for long without water. As such, the stimuli known as "thirst" is activated to tell the body that it needs more water to function properly. Thirst shouldn't be ignored and should be managed in a timely manner or else dehydration may result and health problems may arise if not enough water is consumed.

Heat stroke is a condition wherein the body loses the capacity to handle the heat, resulting in sweating, thirst, loss of electrolytes, weakness, and even fainting. It's during the warmer seasons like summer when the heat steps up a notch. This increases the risk of getting affected by the heat and get dehydrated. Also called as hyperthermia, heat stroke is a dangerous condition that can lead to a number of complications if not treated properly. It's often that the victims of heat stroke are children, young adults, and even animals. Despite the wide range of victims, the management of heat stroke is roughly the same for everyone. Heat stroke often occurs to those who stay out under the sun for too long, especially when it's ill-advised during the summer seasons and in regions where the sun seems to be boiling most of the time, like in the Middle East or in the deserts of Africa or even the wild outback of Australia. It here that those who are not prepared have a higher chance of getting heat stroke.

Heat stroke shouldn't be taken lightly, especially when you're out alone. It can lead to a number of health problems and it may even result in death as the human body can only last for so long without water. Even then, there is more to just drinking water when it comes to battling heat stroke. The management of heat stroke relies on one's determination, patience, and cautiousness when going out under the blazing heat of the sun and coming as prepared to battle the heat of the sunlight.

In this book, you'll be learning on how to manage heat stroke the right way, including its characteristics, its risk factors, the signs and symptoms of heat stroke, ways on how to treat heat stroke, and measures on how to prevent heat stroke from occurring in the first place.

Chapter 1 - What is Heat Stroke?

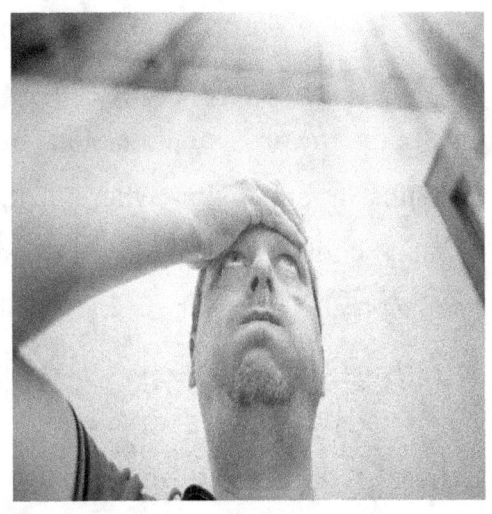

Heat stroke is a condition that can be described as a serious illness that comes from heat. Also called as "hyperthermia", heat stroke results from the excessive rise in one's body temperature, often rising up to or even greater than 40 °C due to a number of factors like excessive exposure to heat, lack of thermoregulatory measures, and insufficient intake of water. Heat stroke is different from a fever as the latter is a physiological response of the body towards an infection, but contains a set point wherein the human body can handle. In heat stroke, that set point or barrier is broken as the temperature rises to new heights which can end up damaging the various vital organs if not treated in the most immediate time.

The term "stroke" in heat stroke is a misnomer since it doesn't involve the interruption of the cerebral blood flow due to a blockage or an incident of hemorrhage. However, this term may relate to the part of the brain that may cease function due to the intense heat that the body experiences and which can lead to the shutdown to some parts of the brain. This may just mean the sudden onset of signs and symptoms of heat stroke which include weakness, dizziness, feeling of fainting, or a loss of consciousness – signs and symptoms that can also be found in stroke.

There are various preventive measures against heat stroke which include drinking plenty of fluids and limiting exposure to excessive heat and humidity, especially during the warmer seasons or staying too long in enclosed and unventilated places like parked cars with sealed windows or a room without a window wherein heat is trapped. Treatment of heat stroke involves the rapid cooling of the body by bringing the temperature close or to the normal through a number of ways.

Heat stroke is considered to be one of the most serious and also one of the most common forms of heat injury. It is considered as a medical emergency as a number of complications can result if proper treatment measures are not instituted to a victim of heat stroke. It is also known to cause damage to the brain and other internal organs if left untreated. While heat stroke is common among those who are 50 years old and above, it can also occur in younger people, particularly those who engage in strenuous physical activities or those who stay under the sun for too long. It should be noted that heat stroke can start from mere heat cramps but can proceed to heat syncope and then heat exhaustion. Heat stroke can also occur even without signs and symptoms of previous heat injury.

Heat stroke can occur after being exposed to an environment with an excessively high temperature, working with dehydration, which can lead to the body's failure to compensate the rise in temperature. It then occurs when the core body temperature exceeds about 40 °C which can cause a number of complications to the central nervous system. Other signs and symptoms of heat stroke may include nausea, vomiting, confusion, weakness, fatigue, diaphoresis, disorientation, loss of consciousness, and even coma.

Risk Factors for Heat Stroke

While heat stroke may sound light, it should be considered as a medical emergency that needs immediate treatment. Heat stroke is a form of hyperthermia or heat-related condition wherein the signs and symptoms can lead to changes in the central nervous system function. Heat stroke can be fatal if emergency measures are not taken. One of the most common causes of heat stroke is dehydration which can prevent sweating, the body's natural defense mechanism to release heat from the body, to occur and lead to the continuing rise of body temperature.

Heat stroke has a number of factors that increase its likelihood of occurring. By knowing these factors, you can prevent the occurrence of heat stroke in the first place. Here are some of the most common risk factors for heat stroke.

Age
Infants and the elderly are particularly at risk for developing

heat stroke because of their susceptibility to temperature changes

Hot or dry seasons

Countries located closer to the equator have increased risk for people to develop heat stroke because of the heat experienced in these regions, especially during the dry seasons.

Prolonged exposure to heat

Exposure to heat for too long increases the likelihood of heat stroke and removal of oneself from the heat is the first measure that should be done.

Excessive physical exertion under the sun

Athletes and workers who stay under the sun and do physical activity are at a greater risk for developing heat stroke.

Insufficient hydration

Dehydration is common among the victims of heat stroke because of inadequate intake of water while under the heat.

Enclosed environment

Enclosed environments like a room without windows or a sealed car don't let heat escape and they don't allow the air to circulate in the environment, increasing the temperature in the area.

Medical conditions

Medical conditions like heart diseases, respiratory diseases, and kidney problems increase the risk for developing heart disease through various factors; for example, a person with renal parenchymal disease may experience the signs and symptoms of heat stroke because of dehydration secondary to their limited intake of fluids for 24 hours.

Use of illegal drugs

Amphetamines, cocaine, LSD, and MDMA can lead to heat stroke or hyperthermia as their adverse effect.

Medications

Some medications increase the likelihood of heat stroke like psychotropic medications, antidepressants, anesthetic agents, and anticholinergic drugs.

Wearing Personal Protective Equipment (PPE)

Heat stroke can occur to those who wear personal protective equipment or PPE. This is because PPEs are enclosed and tight to serve as the protection against the entry of bacteria and viruses, as well as prevent contamination from toxic substances to the person inside the PPE, most often a healthcare practitioner like a doctor or a nurse. This is the reason why most PPE and PPE guidelines advise that those wearing it should only use the PPE for about an hour at most.

Heat stroke should be considered as a medical emergency. While heat stroke may be common in public places like schools, the late intervention could lead to a number of complications that can affect the functions of the central nervous system. Temperature regulation is one of the most basic ways on how to manage heat stroke and it should be instituted on the scene for the heat stroke victim.

Chapter 2 - The Signs and Symptoms of Heat Stroke

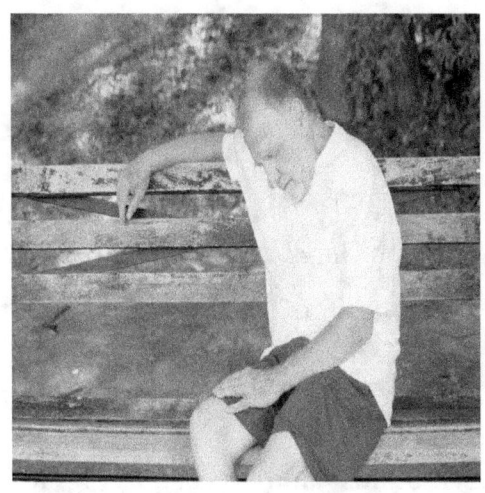

After knowing the basics of heat stroke, it's time to learn on how to recognize this heat injury for what it is depending on its signs and symptoms. Being the most serious form of heat injury, heat stroke has similar signs and symptoms to other heat injuries like heat cramps and heat exhaustion. However, being the most serious type of heat injury, late treatment may result in various complications that can lead to organ failure and even death.

Identifying heat stroke is the first way on how to begin treating it. While heat stroke may sound easy to identify at first glance, you'll need a keen clinical eye to see the signs and symptoms and recognize if it is indeed heat stroke. Signs and symptoms of heat stroke often correlate with similar signs and symptoms of other heat injuries like heat exhaustion and heat cramps.

The hallmark sign of heat stroke is the core body temperature that is more than 40 °C or 105 °F which can cause damage to the central nervous system if not treated in time. Other signs and symptoms are often correlated with the signs and symptoms of dehydration like inability to sweat, loss of electrolytes, and loss of consciousness.Heat injuries are often related to the rise in the body temperature that exceeds the normal range which can lead to neurological damage if not treated in time. Heat stroke is considered to be the most serious form of heat injuries and should be considered as an emergency case.Here are the signs and symptoms that you should watch out if you suspect someone to have heat stroke.

Signs and Symptoms of Heat Stroke:

Fever of more than 40 °C or 105 °F

Throbbing or bounding headache

Dizziness

Lightheadedness

Absence of sweating

Dry and hot skin surface

Weakness

Fatigue

Muscle cramps

Nausea

Vomiting

Rapid heartbeat

Rapid, shallow breathing

Low blood pressure

Confusion

Disorientation

Loss pf consciousness

Seizures

Coma

Heat stroke is considered as a medical emergency. Oftentimes, victims of heat stroke or any other heat injury for that matter are predisposed to getting complications because of delayed seeking of health treatment or the slow interventions of the healthcare team provided that they know the cause of the condition of the patient. While heat stroke is easy to treat during its initial stages, it can be hard to manage once it reaches the emergency threshold that may lead to the damage of the central nervous system or even the dangerous levels of dehydration in some patients which warrant even more aggressive treatment options to resolve. In severe cases of heat stroke, organ failure or even death can occur.

Heat stroke is found to be common among the elderly who live in enclosed environments like apartments or homes without adequate air conditioning or ventilation. Other people who are prone to getting heat stroke include those who don't drink enough water, those who have chronic diseases like heart problems and diabetes mellitus, and those who drink an excessive amount of alcoholic beverages.

The heat index is a strong factor in determining the presence of heat stroke. The heat index is the measurement on how the body feels heat when affected by the relative humidity and the air temperature. For example, an environment with a high percentage of humidity prevents the evaporation of sweat, preventing the body to cool itself during a hot weather.

The risk of getting heat strong further increases when the heat index rises, so it's essential that you know the reported heat index during hot and dry seasons, like during heat waves, and you need to remember that full exposure to the sun during these times may increase the heat index even more, prompting increased precaution to prevent the incidence of heat stroke.

Those living in urban environments may also be prone to getting heat stroke because of a prolonged heat wave. This is because of the stagnant atmospheric conditions and the poor air quality in urban areas wherein air is cannot travel properly and ventilation is often poor because of the closed environments. The "Heat Island Effect" is when the asphalt and the concrete manage to store the heat during the day and gradually releasing it during nighttime, increasing the temperature during the nighttime and increasing the risk of heat stroke if you're not careful.

People living in environments that are open like farmlands in the rural areas are less prone to getting heat stroke because there is better ventilation and adequate airflow in these areas compared to the tightly-knit urban areas. When building homes, it's also encouraged that adequate spacing should be provided between neighboring houses to promote ventilation and airflow, preventing the incidents of heat stroke. Those living in enclosed areas like in urban slums may have an increased risk to develop heat stroke because the environment tends to trap heat throughout the day, especially during the warmer seasons.

Pathophysiology of Heat Stroke

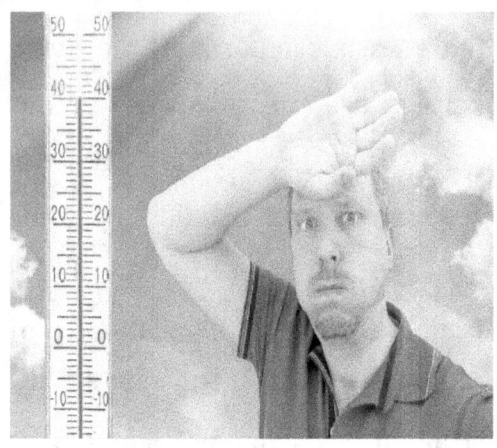

Heat stroke occurs when the core temperature of the body rises above the normal range due to the action of the anterior hypothalamus, the regulating center for temperature located in the brain. A good example is when a viral or bacterial infection occurs and the white blood cells release pyrogens within the blood to combat the infection but have a direct effect on the anterior hypothalamus, raising temperature and eventually causing a fever, as if raising the body's temperature like a thermostat. However, in heat stroke, the body temperature rises beyond the normal range without the change or influence in the heat control centers in the anterior hypothalamus.

Barrier dysfunction and endotoxemia (the presence of toxins often due to bacteria or viruses in the blood) may cause gastrointestinal symptoms in acute exertional heat stroke which may include nausea, vomiting, diarrhea, and even bleeding of the gastrointestinal tract. These toxins can stimulate the cytokines which can result in multi-organ failure if not treated in time.

The metabolic process is the primary function responsible in maintaining a core body temperature within normal range. The anterior hypothalamus in the nervous system than triggers mechanism to manage the heat in the body, either by losing heat like sweating or by generating heat like by shivering or muscle contraction. This region of the brain is found to be filled with neurons that are both insensitive and sensitive to heat and heat changes in the body to determine the set point for the core body temperature. For example, when the body temperature rises beyond the normal range, the electrical impulses to the neurons sensitive to heat increases to compensate. However, when temperature falls below the normal range, the neurons sensitive to the cold get an increased amount of electrical impulses to compensate.

Chapter 3 - Diagnosing Heat Stroke

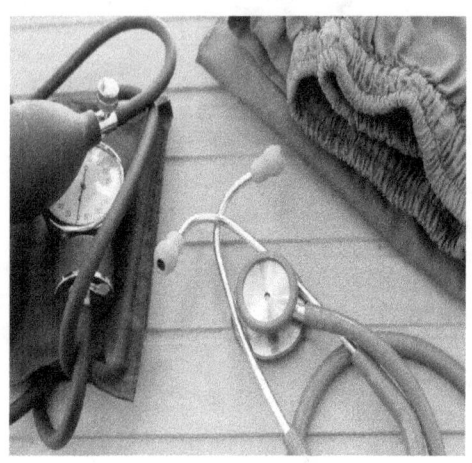

After knowing the basics of heat stroke, it's time to learn on how to recognize this heat injury for what it is depending on its signs and symptoms. Being the most serious form of heat injury, heat stroke has similar signs and symptoms to other heat injuries like heat cramps, heat exhaustion, and dehydration.

Knowing the signs and symptoms of heat stroke is important, but establishing a strong diagnosis of heat stroke may be difficult at times.

As such, there are a number of laboratory tests and diagnostic procedures that can be done, on top of physical assessment to identify the presence of heat stroke.

Heat stroke can be diagnosed through the combination of a high core body temperature and a history that coincides with the incidence of hyperthermia or heat stroke, instead of a fever. This would mean infections from viruses or bacteria are excluded since this may be another medical condition aside from heat stroke.

It is often easy for doctors to detect a heat stroke among patients, but there are also laboratory tests that can be done to confirm their diagnosis. Getting these tests done also rules out other health conditions and strengthen the diagnosis of heat stroke, ensuring that the proper treatment is given. These diagnostic tests can also detect the severity of the heat stroke like detecting the presence of organ damage in the most severe forms of heat stroke.

Serumelectrolytes – checking the serum sodium and potassium are routine blood tests that can identify the presence of dehydration for those suspected to have heat stroke.

Arterialbloodgas – an ABG or arterial blood gas analysis can be done to detect the presence of any damage to the central nervous system for those with heat stroke.

Urinalysis – a urinalysis is done to identify the fluid status for those with heat stroke wherein those who may be dehydrated or have inadequate fluids in their body may have a darker colored urine and the function of the kidneys are also assessed by a simple urinalysis.

Musclefunctiontests – these tests are done to detect any serious damage to the muscle tissue due to heat stroke or any form of heat injury like heat cramps or heat exhaustion.

X-ray – an X-ray may be done to detect any form of organ damage after a prolonged or severe episode of heat stroke.

The most common factor to establish a diagnosis of heat stroke is the presence of an elevated temperature in a hot and humid environment or the presence of exhaustion after doing excessive physical activity under a hot environment without proper hydration. If antipyretics or fever-regulating drugs are administered to the patient and their temperature manages to lower, even if the temperature is still above the normal range, the diagnosis of heat stroke is ruled out.

Chapter 4 - Treatment and Prevention of Heat Stroke

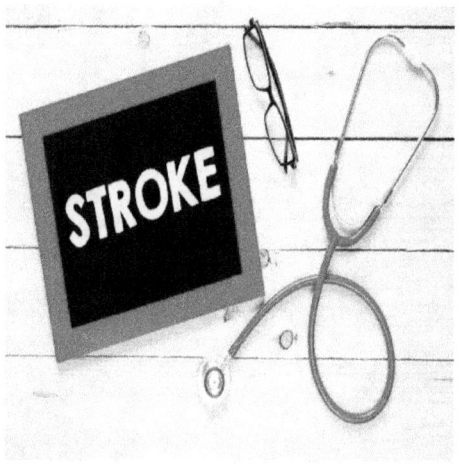

After knowing how to establish a strong diagnosis of heat stroke, it's time to know how to manage heat stroke and institute the emergency measures in order to prevent the various complications that may arise with heat stroke. Providing treatment for heat stroke is often easy during its initial stages because the state of the body is still controllable and the core body temperature can easily be managed through various methods.

Treatment for heat stroke primarily involves the rapid cooling of the body together with the standard resuscitating procedures. Here are the following interventions that you should do when it comes for people who have heat stroke.

Once you see someone fall ill from heat stroke, immediately call for 911 or your local emergency medical team so that the victim may be brought to the hospital.

Move the person to a cooler area, whether indoors or under the shade to help lower the temperature of the body faster.

Clothing should be removed to promote heat loss and lower body temperature through passive cooling.

Bathing in cold water is one of the active ways to cool down someone with a heat stroke.

A hyperthermia vest can be applied to promote adequate reduction of heat of the body.

Don't cover someone in wet towels or clothes as these can act as a form of insulation and further increase the core body temperature even further.

Apply a cool compress to the head, the neck, the groin, or the torso to help cool down the temperature of the victim.

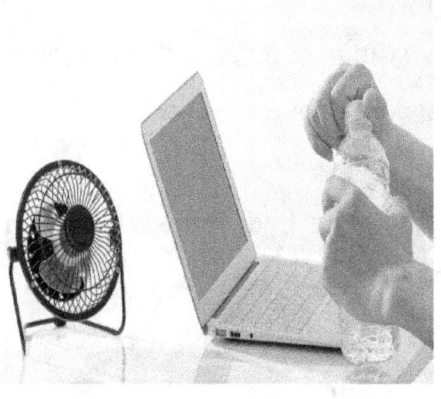

Turning on a fan or air conditioning can allow the evaporation of water and help in cooling down the body for the victim of heat stroke.

Immersing yourself in a tub of cool water is a widely accepted method of cooling for those with heat stroke, though it may need the help of other people and the victim should be monitored throughout the immersion therapy; this method is avoided if the person is unconscious, but if there is no other alternative of cooling the victim rapidly, their head must be kept above the water.

Adequate hydration is a must if the person is conscious to ensure that the heat stroke victim does not choke while drinking.

Drinking sports drinks can help in both hydration and restoring the lost electrolytes in cases of heat stroke.

In excessive physical activity, a loss of electrolytes can occur and drinking more water can worsen the condition due to *dilutional hyponatremia* wherein the ratio of water far exceeds the amount of sodium in the body; instead, drinking sports drinks that are filled with electrolytes.

If the person is unconscious, starting an intravenous drip may be done to provide adequate hydration and provide supplementary electrolytes.

If a heat stroke victim goes into cardiac arrest, cardiopulmonary resuscitation or CPR should be done immediately.

Preventing Heat Stroke

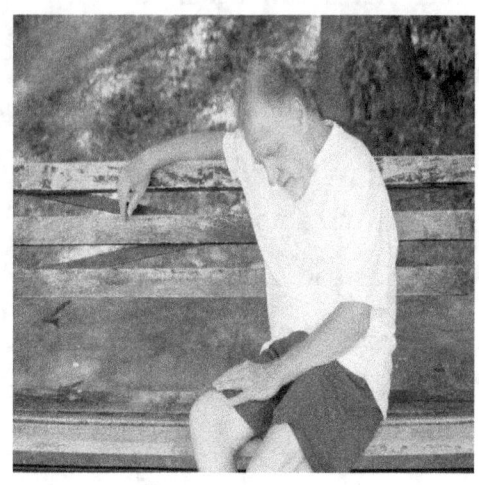

Preventing heat stroke from happening in the first place is possible. The risk of getting heat stroke can be reduced by instituting a number of precautions to prevent the overheating of the body and prevent dehydration. Here are the following measures that you can follow to prevent the incidence of heat stroke.

Wear light and loose-fitting clothes to promote ventilation, promote the evaporation of sweat, and prevent the excessive buildup of heat, especially during the warmer seasons.

Wearing wide-brimmed hats can help protect your head and neck from the heat of the sun.

Drink plenty of cool liquids to compensate and replace for the fluids that you've lost through sweating and physical activity.

Avoid exercising during noontime or anytime when the heat of the sun is at its maximum since this will promote excessive heat buildup.

Don't stay in confined spaces like automobiles or enclosed rooms without adequate ventilation or air-conditioning as the heat becomes trapped and the temperature of the body rises without adequate ventilation.

Avoid drinking alcoholic beverages and drinks that contain caffeine since they promote the excretion of fluids from the body, promoting dehydration and preventing the water buildup in the body that is essential in cooling down the core body temperature during the heat.

Cool off using a fan or wetting yourself with damp sheets on your neck, face, arms, and legs, especially during the warmer seasons.

Take a cool shower or bath to cool down if you're outdoors and nowhere near a shaded area.

Apply high quality sunscreen – with at least an SPF level of 15 – to protect yourself from sunburns and reduce the amount of heat that your body receives from the heat of the sun.

Be careful in some medications as they can raise the core body temperature and worsen the episode of a heat stroke.

Don't leave anyone inside a parked car, whether if it's your child or a pet, since the temperature within this enclosed space can rise to the extreme and it can even lead to the death of children and pets if left alone even as little as 10 minutes.

Avoid physical activity during the hottest part of the day as this can only contribute to heat exhaustion and heat stroke.

Try to get used to the level of heat in your area and you'll eventually handle the heat without having troubles and this will make you resistant to the heat and prevent episodes of heat stroke.

Chapter 5 - Heat Stroke Facts

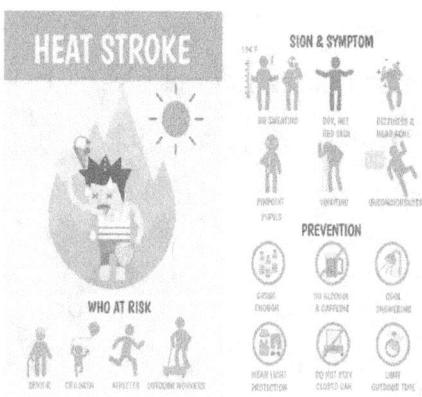

Knowing the various treatment options for heat stroke, you'll probably realize at how easy it is to apply first aid to a victim of heat stroke. You'll also notice at how easy it is to prevent heat stroke from occurring in the first place. After knowing the basics of heat stroke like its signs and symptoms, diagnosing heat stroke, and treating heat stroke, there are still some facts that you should know about it. As a summary, here are some heat stroke facts.

Heat stroke is the most serious form of heat injury, standing alongside heat cramps and heat exhaustion.

Heat stroke is a form of hyperthermia, described as an abnormal rise in the core body temperature without the presence of other factors like bacterial or viral infections.

Heat stroke is considered as a medical emergency and it can be deadly if not treated in time.

Dehydration often accompanies heat stroke which further aggravates the condition.

Heat stroke can be diagnosed through the recognition of the signs and symptoms of a victim who is exposed to an excessively warm or hot environment.

Heat stroke treatment involves cooling down the victim which is an essential step in preventing the complications that may arise from heat stroke.

Notify an emergency service immediately if you suspect someone to have heat stroke.

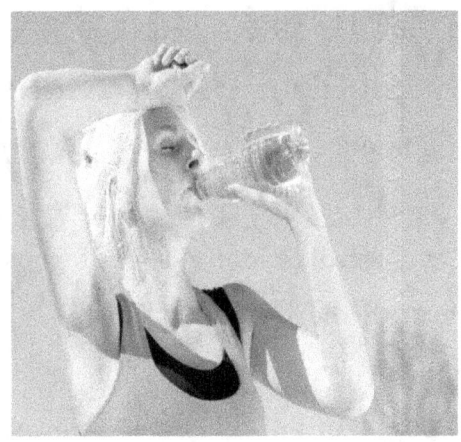

Adequate hydration and doing physical activities in hot and humid environments are key points in preventing the occurrence of heat stroke in the first place.

Groups who are at risk of getting heat stroke include infants, younger children, athletes, the elderly, outdoor workers, and those who have a pre-existing chronic medical condition.

Don't leave children or pets inside a parked car because even in moderate weather conditions, the temperature can rise above the normal range and cause heat stroke for those inside the car.

Fortunately, the prognosis for heat stroke is often good. Once emergency treatment measures are instituted, the outlook for victims of heat stroke is often for the better. Dehydration is managed through the adequate ingestion of fluids, either by oral intake or by intravenous fluids. Supplying electrolytes through IV fluids and drinks is also essential so that complications won't arise from heat stroke.

After recovering from heat stroke, victims can become more sensitive to higher temperatures for a few more weeks. Because of this, it's advised that physical activity outdoors and staying outdoors for too long during a hot day should be avoided until your attending physician tells you that's it is okay for you to resume your usual daily activities.

CONCLUSION

Heat stroke is one of the most common medical emergencies during the summer seasons and in those regions particularly close to the equator. The scorching heat of the sun is the primary culprit to this condition, raising the core body temperature above normal and leading to a number of signs and symptoms that indicate a medical emergency that needs immediate medical treatment. If not treated in time, heat stroke can be fatal and other complications like multi-organ failure, coma, or even death can occur.

Because of how common it is, it's important that you know how to identify the signs and symptoms of heat stroke and how to manage it, even if you're not a medical practitioner. While it may be considered as an emergency case, heat stroke can be easy to manage and it is even easier to prevent from happening in the first place.

The primary goal of treating heat stroke is cooling down the victim's core body temperature through a number of ways which include evaporation, mechanical cooling, conduction of heat, and active cooling like immersing the heat stroke victim in cool water. All it takes is a calm mind and sharp decision making to ensure that the heat stroke victim gets the treatment that he or she needs.

Aside from helping those who may be a victim of heat stroke, you can also use what you've learned so far to help yourself in preventing and managing heat stroke if you suspect that you've become a victim yourself.

All you need to do is be calm, be cool, and stay sharp.